The Magic of Pomegranates

For Health and Beauty

I0422903

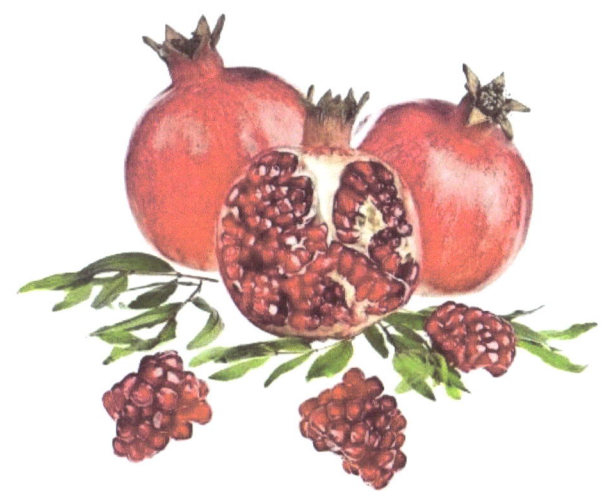

Dueep J Singh
Natural Remedy Series
Mendon Cottage Books

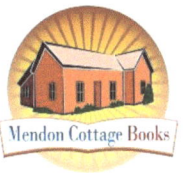

JD-Biz Publishing
Download Free Books!

http://MendonCottageBooks.com

Disclaimer

The information is this book is provided for informational purposes only. It is not intended to be used and medical advice or a substitute for proper medical treatment by a qualified health care provider. The information is believed to be accurate as presented based on research by the author.

The contents have not been evaluated by the U.S. Food and Drug Administration or any other Government or Health Organization and the contents in this book are not to be used to treat cure or prevent disease.

The author or publisher is not responsible for the use or safety of any diet, procedure or treatment mentioned in this book. The author or publisher is not responsible for errors or omissions that may exist.

Warning

The Book is for informational purposes only and before taking on any diet, treatment or medical procedure, it is recommended to consult with your primary health care provider.

Our books are available at

1. Amazon.com

2. Barnes and Noble

3. Itunes

4. Kobo

5. Smashwords

6. Google Play Books

Table of Contents

Introduction

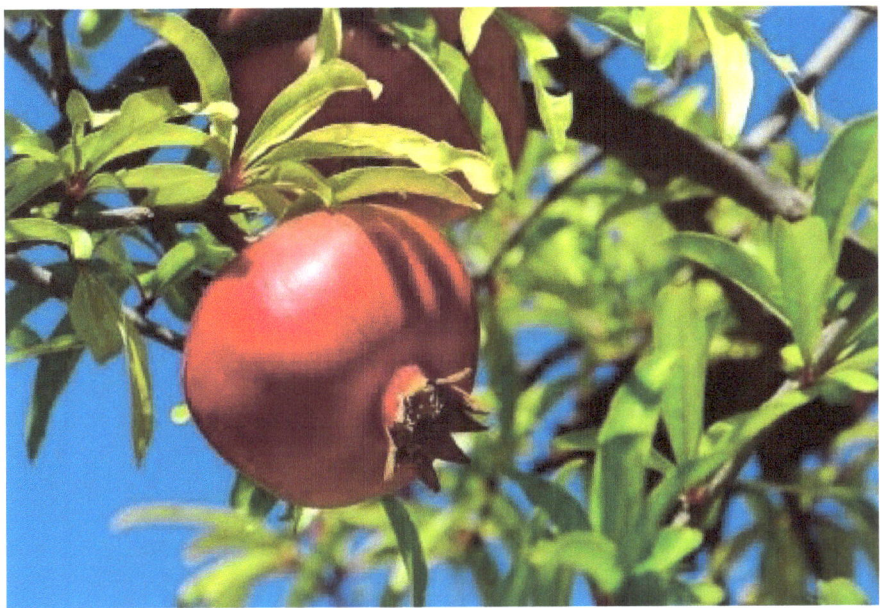

In this book of our **Magic** Series, the author is proud to bring pomegranates to the readers' notice. Since ancient times, pomegranates have been an integral part of ancient medicine and natural remedies. Pomegranates have been called the Poor man's doctor, because since ancient times, man has been curing himself with spices, fruits, herbs and nuts.

That is why people of the 21st century are coming back to nature and looking for natural remedies, which are going to cure them of diseases and ailments. Chemical-based drugs may heal you very well on a short-term basis, but they are going to have an everlasting long-term effect on your body. On the other hand, fruits and vegetables as well as herbs are going to heal your body naturally, while making sure that you do not suffer from any sort of side effects. This is the reason why the magic series are going to tell you all about the wonderful medical and beauty enhancing benefits of different herbs, spices, fruit, vegetables and flowers.

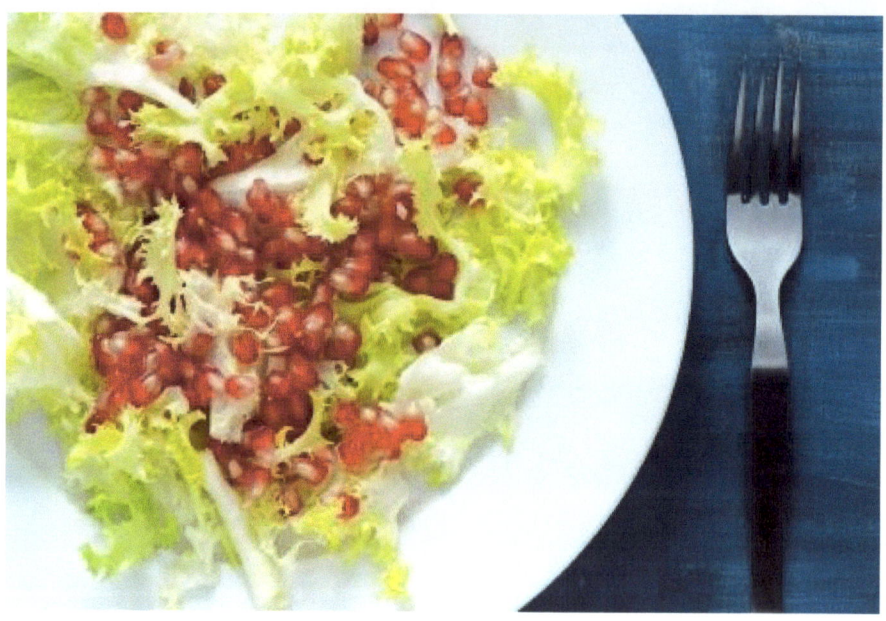

Ancient medical treatises in Egypt and Persia consider pomegranates to be a powerhouse of good health. That is because they thought that this fruit could cure people of many ills. The Latin name for pomegranate is Punica granatum. One wonders whether the Romans fought the Punic wars with Carthage, to rule over lands where they could get pomegranates, because after all, everybody knows that the Roman emperors ransomed Kings for black pepper, exotic fruit and other spices.

According to ancient treatises, the pomegranate had the power to purify your blood, which would mean that your skin would not suffer from any sort of skin ailments, including pimples or boils. Also, when I was talking about pomegranates, with an ancient naturopath, he told me that sages of ancient time used to use pomegranate seeds to enhance brain power and vision, get rid of adema, renew the mineral resources needed for keeping our body working properly and reduce urinary inconsistency.

In fact, he handed me some pomegranate seeds, mixed up with rock salt, to make me feel hungry. [I had lost my appetite, because of illness and also due to stress.] He said that that activated the stomach and made it do its job properly and naturally. It worked. So if you have a continuous access to pomegranates, lucky, lucky you!

The pomegranate peels are going to keep you beautiful. The pomegranate seeds' juice is going to keep you healthy, both externally and internally.

Pomegranates for Beauty and Skincare

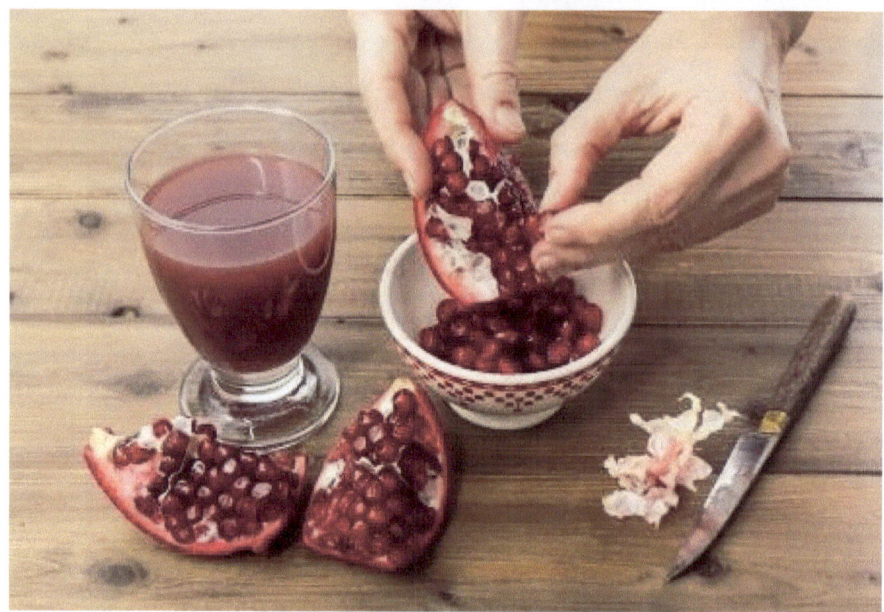

Pomegranates have been used since ancient times to enhance the beauty of the skin. I read in a translation of an ancient book, that ancient Egyptians and Greeks used to use pomegranates, not only for enhancing their skins, but Julius Caesar used the dried skins, as well as hot walnut shells as a depilatory. How painful! Nevertheless, all you have to do is to try out this recipe to get a beautiful skin complexion and texture.

Pomegranate peels for beauty

Collect the skins of ripe pomegranates – wild pomegranates are best for this, because their fruit are more potent and powerful. I did not manage to find that same sort of power in hybrid plants. Dry these shells in the sun. If you manage to dry citrus fruit skins, like oranges, lemons, and other citrus fruits at the same time, you are going to add even more power to your beauty masks. After you have found them all dried and shriveled, just grind them into a fine powder   either together, or on their own. Put them in a glass bottle and mix them with the powder of dried gooseberries – Emblica Officianalis-. In India, this paste is normally used all over the body, as a scrub with rosewater, before you have a bath.

In all my magic series, you are going to find a recipe on how to make rosewater. As the series are to make sure that you do not spend lots of money in buying chemical-based lotions and potions from the market, it is much better to make natural products right at home. For that, you just need to have access to the right ingredients and some free time in which you can make these products. I often do that in an afternoon. This rosewater is going to be the base of all your masks, irrespective of the ingredients you use, whether fruit, spices, honey, or any other beauty enhancing product. You can also use the rosewater to flavor any of your desserts, with the aroma of exotic roses, the perfume of the East.

Pomegranate peels facemasks

Pomegranate peels facemasks have been in use since millenniums, by Egyptians, Persians, Greeks, Chinese, Indians, and any other ancient civilization of which the women knew how to beautify themselves naturally.

These skins were collected and sun-dried in the shade in the summer. Then they were powdered very finely, and then filtered. Half a teaspoonful of pomegranate peels powder and half a teaspoonful of orange peel powder, along with some exotic rosewater, some honey and almond oil and some fullers earth is going to make an excellent facemask. If you want to use pomegranate peels powder as a scrub, in your shower, leave out the fuller's earth. Instead, add oatmeal. This is the life with youthful, silky smooth and blemish free, healthy skin.

Use this pomegranate peel mask at least twice a week, or whenever you feel like indulging yourself.

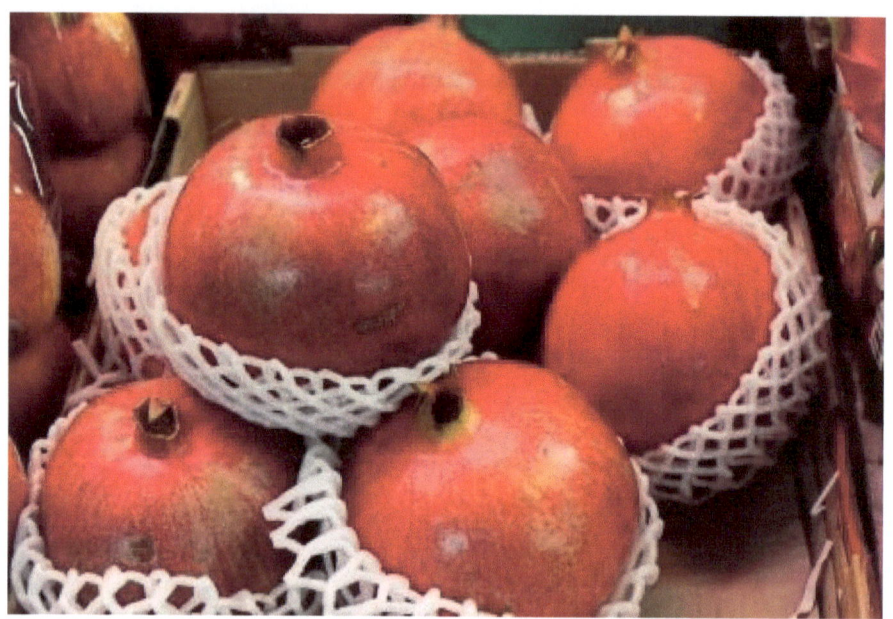

How to make Rose water (Gulab Jal)

Rosewater is normally available in markets at exorbitant prices, but in India, anybody with access to the red rose - Rosa Damascena, - used in India and Iran or Rosa Centifolia which is used in Bulgaria, and Germany-and a little bit of time enjoys making Rosewater at home. This Rosewater is used in cosmetics, as well as in cookery to impart the flavor of the Rose to your meal or to your skin.

Ingredients needed- 1 Cup Rose petals - 12 to 14 flowers.

2 cups water

Lots of ice.

A huge cooking pan - pan number one - with lid in which another pan - pan number two - can be placed comfortably.

Rosewater is just a matter of distillation. Put a wire stand in pan number one, on which you are going to stand the other pan number two. The condensed Rosewater is going to fall into pan number two.

Place the petals at the bottom of the pan number one. Now, cover the petals with water. Place pan number two on the wire stand. Now take the lid and place it upside down on pan number one, thus effectively covering the Rose petals, pan number two and the water. The Rose water is going to condense when you place the blocks and chunks of ice on the inverted lid.

You are going to have a cupful of precious distilled Rosewater, after 25 minutes of slow steaming of the Rose petals.

Precautions - remember to have enough of water to cover the Rose petals. Also, it should not be of such a large quantity, that it displaces the wire stand.

This cooled water is now pure Rosewater. Place it in a sterilized glass bottle. Use it to your heart's content. You may see a little bit of oil swimming over the surface of the water. This is Rose oil, and is even more precious. So if you used lots of petals in a larger pan, you may find even more Rose oil.

This method is for all those people who use a pressure cooker while cooking food. In fact, it is a common way to cook food in Asian kitchens, instead of using the microwave.

You would need water, petals, a pressure cooker and a long thin pipe which it does not melt, when subjected to heat.

Put the water and the petals in the pressure cooker and cover it. Now cover the thin pipe with wet cloth in order to keep it cool. Attach this pipe on the lid of the pressure cooker where you normally attach the weight. Allow the petals to cook slowly, they seem to build up, go through the cooled pipe and collect in a utensil. I tried this way too, but I find the ice on the lid one easier!

So now that you know all about how to make rosewater, and you know how to use it to make a pomegranates skin mask for your body, it is going to get rid of blemishes, dullness, shallowness in your skin and other skin ailments naturally and leave your skin silky smooth and glowing.

Wrinkles

Reduce wrinkles by drinking and applying pomegranate juice.

If you have a pomegranate tree in a garden near by, you do not have to worry about any sort of skin ailments, ever. In fact, if you are suffering from wrinkles, apply a mixture of powdered pomegranate seeds mixed up with sesame oil to the affected area and massage it twice a day. Throw away your antiwrinkle creams, right now. You may also want to get rid of wrinkles by massaging your body with mustard oil before you have a shower. Well, let me admit it, mustard oil pongs. That is why this massage is normally done by athletes every evening or by health conscious people on Sunday, so that they can get rid of that smell with a hot shower afterwards.

Pimples

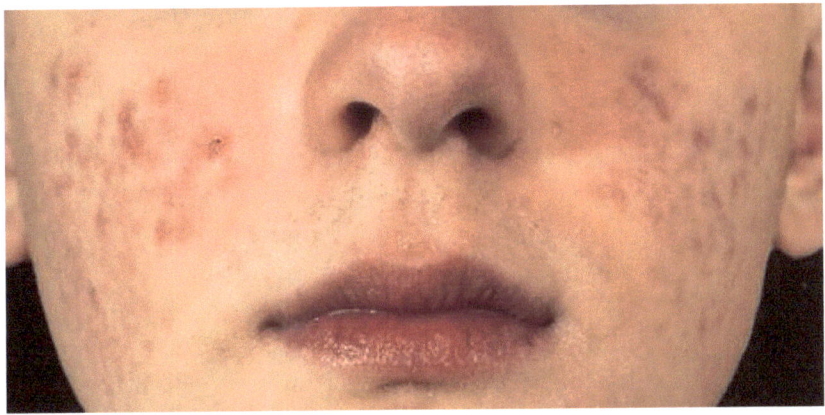

Believe it or not, pimples can be cured really well with the help of pomegranate root bark, as long as you do not interfere with them by scratching them, or trying to get rid of the accumulated sebum under the skin surface. This is going to scar your skin.

Make a mixture of powdered pomegranate root bark with water. Apply it on the affected areas to dry up the pimples.

Put some blended   gooseberry fruit pulp and fresh pomegranate seeds in some water overnight. Then the next morning, make up a mixture of this paste with more water and wash your face with it. The gooseberries are going to dry out the pimples, and the pomegranate's good for disinfecting your skin.

These are the things that you need to avoid, if you are suffering from pimples or acne. Sore items, fried items, red pepper, hot spices, chocolate and tea. These are just some of the contributing factors, which may cause an acne flareup.

Patchy skin – Leukoderma

Are you suffering from skin patches or leukoderma? This is a distressing disease, in which you may find the melanin content under the surface of your skin disappearing. This leaves your skin surface completely white in patches. It almost feels like as if you have burnt your skin. People are still researching on the reasons for these patches, but the ancients considered it to, because due to toxin buildup and other problems in the system.

You may lighten the skin patches by applying a mixture of powdered pomegranate peelss in almond oil on these patches. This is going to encourage the skin to grow more melanin.

Pomegranates for curing ailments and diseases

In ancient Indian medical treatises, the pomegranate has been called *Dadhim*. The great sage Charaka said in 300 BC in his compendium of Charaka-"man is responsible for all his illnesses, because he does not know how to regulate his food and drink. He overeats on rich and greasy food, and thus causes a lot of illnesses in his body due to the accumulated toxins." This is absolutely true, even 2300 years down the line. We are not very careful about what we eat, and that is the reason why our bodies are subject to so many ailments, especially chronic diseases. In ancient times, the ancients did not advise the eating of meat and spicy food. He continues that *Dadhim* is a powerful weapon to get rid of all these diseases. He advocates exercise, along with 10 to 50 seeds of the pomegranate every day, to get rid of any sort of ailment.

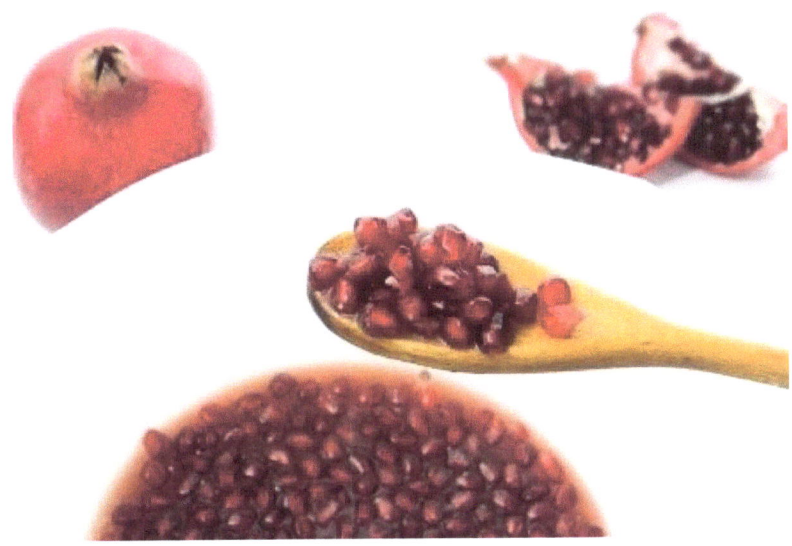

Now, why are we not using this advice? Easy, we enjoy our food, we enjoy eating plenty of delicious, spicy, sour, sweet, hot, rich, vegetarian, and nonvegetarian food. Besides this, we do not stint on alcoholic drinks, because eating and drinking good food and wine is one of the great pleasures of our lives. So if you have a pomegranate tree, in your house, well, you know that you have the natural way in which you can prevent yourself from getting really ill. Pomegranates are very much in demand, and are grown in Western Europe, the Middle East, India, Java and Sumatra, Thailand, Burma, China, and other tropical and dry areas of the world. I would suggest pomegranate farming in California, because the climate there is totally suitable to the growth of a pomegranate tree.

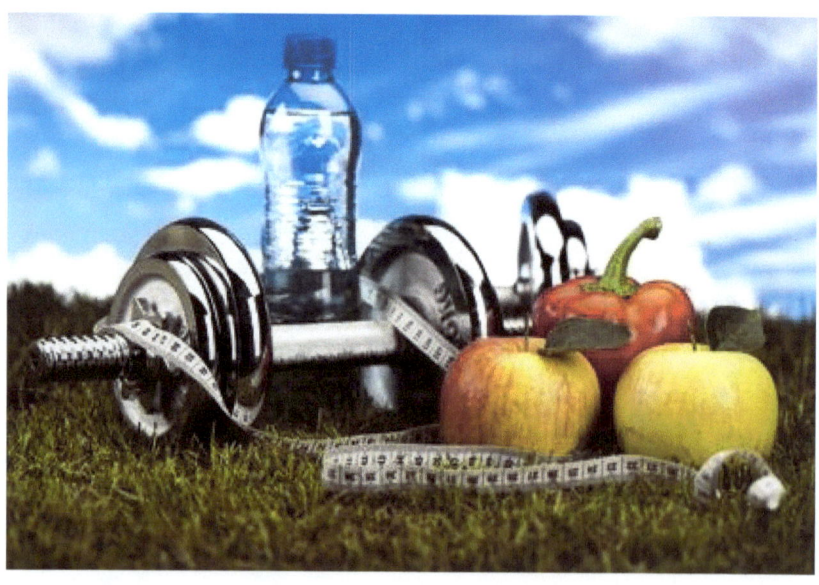

Stay healthy with fruit,vegetables , exercise, and plenty of fresh air.

Look for pomegranate plants, which are not hybrids. If you have a wild pomegranate growing somewhere near you, good, because these plants grown without the help of organic fertilizer and the hand of man are going to give you seeds and fruit, which are going to keep you and your family healthy.

Pomegranate juice has been used in the East, for a long time to get rid of constipation, and also to get your digestive system moving. The pomegranate seed has a mixture of tastes, sweet, sour, a little bit of bitterness and even a tangy flavor. In Chinese medicine, pomegranates were used by the ancients to get rid of dangerous toxins, and to strengthen the mind, heart, body and soul. The idea of ancient medicine is to put the body in harmony with all the elements in it, and around it. The pomegranate does that for you.

Cure for obesity

Did you know that pomegranate have been used since ancient times to prevent excess weight. Of course, those people used to exercise regularly, but you can try these remedies to get rid of that excess weight. Drink 4 tablespoons full of pomegranate juice with 2 tablespoons full of the juice of sacred basil, also known as tulasi once every day. This is going to make your metabolism work properly.

 Inversely, if you are extremely thin, and want to add some weight naturally, add 1 tablespoon full of lemon and horseradish juice to pomegranate juice and drink a glass full of it. Drink this juice Once every day. This is going to help you increase weight naturally and look healthier. In fact, I found that I managed to put on weight – being very badly anorexic and underweight until my 40s – by just drinking pomegranate juice with rock salt. Like I said, my sluggish metabolism woke up and started working just wonderfully.

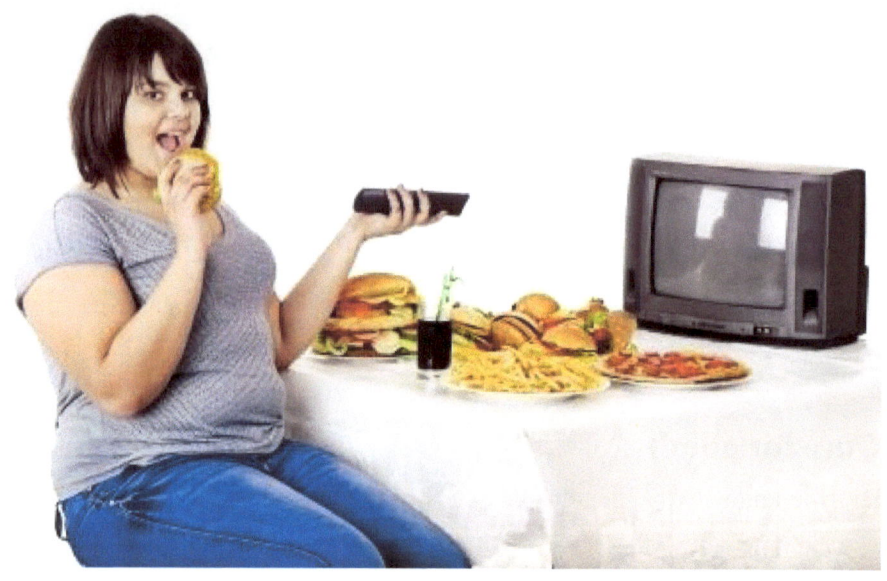

Eating junk food does not help to control or manage obesity.

Insomnia

This is for people who are suffering from chronic insomnia. Believe me, it works. You are never going to find yourself watching the clock. That is because you are going to make a mixture of 10 g aniseed and 10 g pomegranate seeds. Now, boil it in 1 L water until it is reduced to one fourth the amount. Filter it, and put it in a bottle. Now you are going to empty this full bottle by drinking of it twice a day with just one pinch of rock salt. Do this until you find yourself sleeping like a baby, the moment you intend to sleep. It is going to take 4 to 5 days, unless there is something seriously wrong with your system. Stop eating rich and indigestible as well as fried food or alcohol for dinner. Also, avoid stress. Try some physical exercise throughout the day, instead of being a slouch- potato[1] in front of your computer.

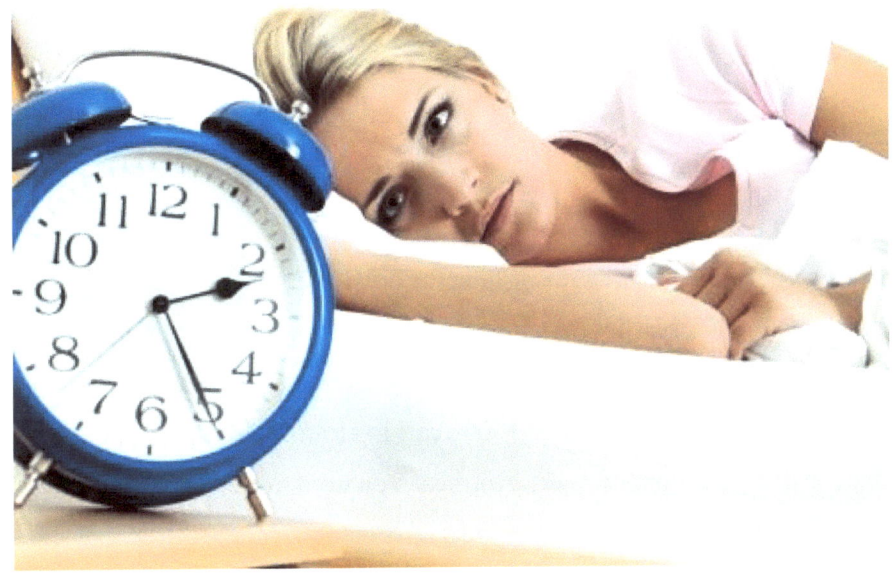

---

[1] This term has been coined by me for global usage, as opposed to couch potato, scrunched up in front of the TV. I am a confirmed sedentary slouch- potato, are you one?

Drink a mixture of pomegranate juice and lemon juice once a day. You may also want to add one spoon of green coriander juice to this mixture. Coriander juice really makes one feel sleepy.

Put one teaspoonful of aniseed in half a cup water and boil it. Now add this water into the juice of pomegranate and drink it up. Even chronic insomniacs are going to say that this remedy works, when drunk once a day. Ancient people brought down this remedy to us, and I do not know how aniseed and pomegranate work together, but I do know that it is effective.

Now this is the recipe, which I like, because it has dried ginger in it. Dried powder ginger 5 g added to warm pomegranate juice. Drink it up and good night, sleep tight! You are definitely also not going to suffer from any throat problem at night, thanks to this dried ginger.

Pomegranate peel Tooth powder

I saw an old lady in a village crushing the dried skin of a pomegranate , a little bit of alum, powdered walnut shells, 10 g, cinnamon with finely powdered rock salt and making it into a fine tooth powder. This recipe has been in existence for more than 1000 years to clean teeth, both from inside and outside. The alum prevents pyorrhea. You need to clean your teeth, morning and evening, with this powder. According to her, she said that she did not know anything about toothpastes, because her ancestors used to use this mixture to keep their teeth shining, healthy, and trouble-free. The proof of the pudding was that she was in her 70s and had still not lost a tooth in her head.

 So try out this tooth powder right now. I did some innovations in this recipe, especially when I noticed   bleeding gums – I added some mustard oil to this tooth powder, before I brushed my teeth and gums with that, believe it or not, the gums stopped bleeding in 2 days and they have not bled since. But then, mustard oil and salt is a good combination to which you can prevent any sort of tooth infection in your teeth. Nevertheless, mustard oil is very smelly, and that is why you may want to use it with care, especially when you are going out. Use mouthwash afterwards. What about the oily feel, after you have brushed your teeth with mustard oil? That can be removed by washing your mouth out with salt water and then giving your teeth, a brisk rub with a clean cloth. Behold, the mirrors beaming and gleaming out at the world.

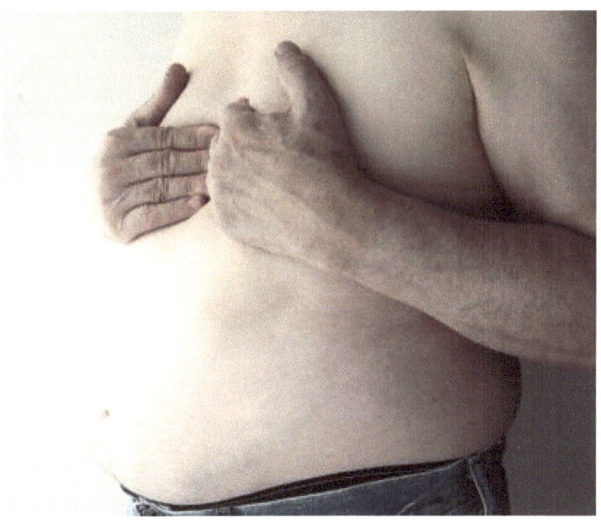

Ill health caused due to infections and excessive Body fat may also give rise to edema.

Edema

This swelling is normally caused when you have some sort of infection inside you, or if your body is dehydrated. That means that there is water retention going on somewhere. Whenever I find myself suffering from any sort of swelling, anytime, I balance the electrolytes in my body by drinking a mixture of coconut water along with pomegranate juice. This is a guaranteed effective remedy. Stop eating tomatoes, oily foods, and spices, if you are suffering from this ailment.

Joint Pain- Gout

According to ancient Ayurveda, this is normally caused when your joints begin to swell up and start causing you pain. This normally takes place as you grow older. In the beginning, you may not enjoy eating your meals, and you feel thirsty. Apart from that, you find yourself with digestive problems. Your joints start aching.

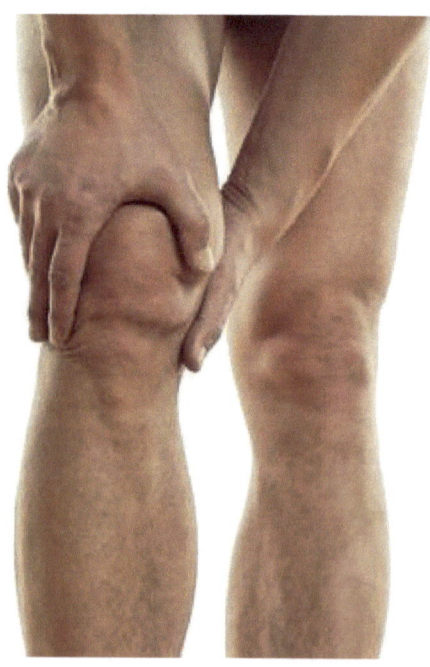

Here are some foods which are going to help you cure joint pain – fenugreek, aubergine, bitter gourd, dates, apples and papayas. In fact, this is also very beneficial to cure gout. Try making a chutney of 10 to 15 pomegranate seeds with one clove of garlic. Eat this with one glass of hot water once every day until you find yourself much better.

This same naturopath told me that massaging the affected areas of people suffering from a stroke or even paralysis with sesame or mustard oil in which you have burnt dried pomegranate seeds and dried pomegranate peels is considered to be a good way in which you can get the muscles moving properly and back to healing. This is going to be a long process, but doing this massage 3 times a day can help heal the affected area. Honestly speaking, nobody has the time to do that in this Hurry worry world, except somebody who really cares for the patient. If the paralysis does not go away, make sure that you have the patient under the proper medical jurisdiction of a qualified, experienced doctor. Do not go in for self-proclaimed know it alls and quack remedies. These natural cures are external, so along with the internal medicine, you are going to have the knowledge and assurance that you are helping in keeping the stroke or paralysis affected muscles and area, mobile and moving through massage.

Tummy Aches

Why do people suffer so often from tummy aches? That means that they have some digestion problems. If your food is not assimilated properly – after digestion – in the rest of your body, it is going to cause problems throughout your system. Tummy aches are extremely common especially when we eat something which does not suit our systems. I am going to tell you a very delicious remedy, which is very common in India and in other parts of the East. It is called a digestive powder or churna. We normally eat

1 tablespoon of this after every heavy meal. There is absolutely no chance of us suffering from indigestion, constipation, or even any other digestion related problems, thanks to the power of pomegranate seeds.

Pomegranate Digestive Special Powder

Collect hundred grams of dried pomegranate seeds, 50 g of jaggery/molasses/crystallized sugar, also known as mishri-5 g, black pepper, 1 g dried ginger, one pinch of asafoetida, 5 g black salt [this is different from rock salt and sea salt. This is black in color and has less sodium content. It also has a sharper spicier taste.] 1 teaspoon cumin seeds, 1 teaspoon fennel seeds, 2 teaspoons bishops weed. Grind them all together into a powder. These are normally made into small beans and sold in the market , as *anardana churna* in India.

I saw something similar sold in the markets of Thailand and Malaysia, with pomegranate seeds, pepper, ginger and black salt. So this digestive powder is indigenous in the East, and is very popular, it seems. I normally put it in a glass bottle and eat a teaspoonful with warm water after every meal. It is yummy. You can also eat it 1st thing in the morning with warm water. This mixture of spices keeps your digestive system healthy. It also makes sure that you do not suffer from ulcers.

I have noticed that if I eat this last thing at night, it is going to clear out my system, early in the morning. So, who needs constipation remedies.

You may also want to get rid of stomachache, by making a chutney of green pomegranate leaves, 2 cloves, a pinch of asafoetida, 2 tablespoons full of bishops weed and 2 tablespoons full of cumin seeds with 3 tablespoons full of lemon juice. Eat this chutney, with your meals twice or thrice a day and see, hey, no tummy ache at all. What fun! We can eat heartily, we can eat what we want, and what is allowed, as long as we have these digestive yummy recipes with us.

Diminished digestive capacity

Believe it or not, there are people who cannot digest even the smallest amounts of food. That means that they are not going to feel hungry after a while. You may find yourself losing your appetite, and finding yourself suffering from this low digestive power of your system, if you are mentally and emotionally disturbed. This is the side effect of stress. And this is a vicious circle, because if you cannot digest your food properly, you are not going to feel hungry.

Try this remedy-I have found it a really good stress buster and also, it improves the appetite of all those people, who have stopped eating because of stress.

Make up a mixture of one pinch of asafoetida and 4 teaspoons full of bishops weed and black salt. Eat one spoon of this mixture with pomegranate juice daily. You are going to find your appetite coming back with a roar within 7 to 15 days. You can also try out this remedy. Drink a glass full of pomegranate juice with ginger and black salt in it, after lunch and dinner. This is delicious. This is also a good detoxifier.

The Spicy Pomegranate Special!

I cannot resist this tasty drink. It is 4 teaspoons full of pomegranate juice with the juice of half a lemon with black salt after lunch and dinner. I use this particular combination as an appetizer enhancer and in fact, whenever I go out to my favorite juice shop in the city, I ask him to make up a glass full of pomegranate juice with ginger, lemon juice, black salt and pepper. He now calls it the Spicy Pomegranate Special!

Indigestion

All of us have suffered from indigestion one time or the other throughout our lives. Indigestion may also be accompanied with tummy ache, especially when we have been eating lots of rich indigestible food and then going straight to sleep without any mild walking exercise in between.

Believe it or not, if you suffer a lot from indigestion, you are going to find yourself weakening day by day. That is because the essential nutrients which are required to keep your system working properly are not being assimilated into your system. They cannot affect your system beneficially. So that is the reason why the ancients say – eat regular meals, at regular times, and also eat a little less than what your hunger demands.

Try this natural remedy, which I found out was very effective. Hundred grams pomegranate juice, hundred grams carrot juice and 150 grams spinach juice. Make up this juice concoction, add a little bit of lemon juice and ginger juice to it, and a little bit of black salt and pepper to make it more palatable. Put it in the fridge, and drink it twice a day. 2 days of this juice mixture, and you are going to find your digestive system waking up and taking notice of the world around it, wonderfully.

You can also try half a cup of pomegranate juice, with 2 spoons of honey and onion juice, once a day. This is what the oldsters who I know swear is the best way to keep their digestive system strong. Also, you may want to try this recipe – one spoon horseradish juice, 4 spoons pomegranate juice, 2 spoons lemon juice, one pinch, rocksalt, pepper to taste, and ¼ teaspoon bishops weed powder – nice and yummy. Drink this down, once a day and get rid of indigestion, even if it is chronic.

Acidity

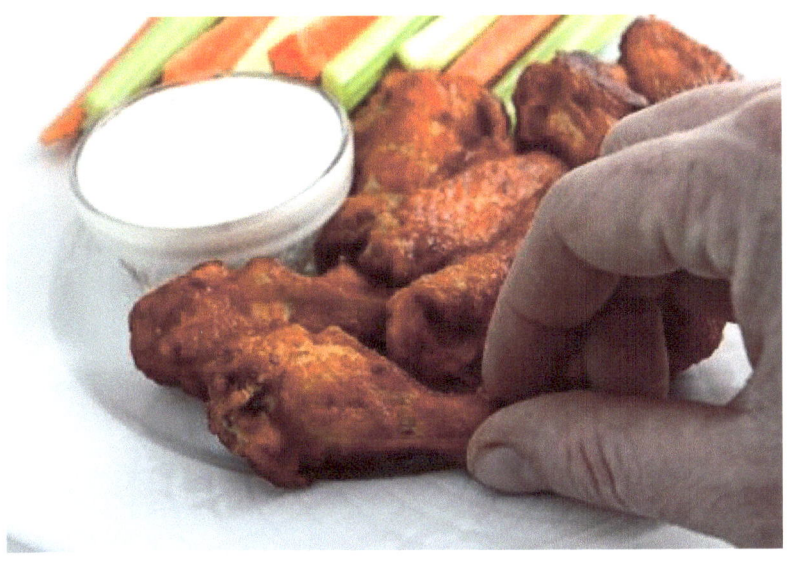

Hot greasy spicy food in summer will cause acidity.

Are you suffering from acidity? This normally occurs when the acid content in your stomach increases, and starts to have an harmful effect on your digestive system. Also, people suffering from acidity are going to be more prone to ulcers, because the acid is going to attack the intestinal lining. Stop eating fatty foods, spicy foods, rice, fried foods and also foods made of processed wheat flour like breads, etc.. Chew your food properly so that it gets mixed properly with saliva.

Take 15 g of dried pomegranate peelss and 2 cloves. Put them in one cup of water and boil them until you have half a cup of water. Add half a cup of carrot juice to this mixture. Drink it down. This is the way in which you are going to cure acidity properly.

You may also want to try out this mixture – 2 tablespoons each of pomegranate and horseradish juice in which you add one pinch of rock salt and a pinch of ground bishops weed. This juice mixture is excellent for curing acidity and getting your system working properly again.

Parasites in your tummy – do you remember the time when grandmother fed you with 4 red potatoes, liberally sprinkled with black pepper, 1st thing in the morning to get rid of the worms and parasites in your tummy? This ancient remedy is still in vogue, in the East, and 3 to 4 days of this drastic treatment gets rid of all the worms and parasites which have dared to set up house in your digestive system. I am giving you another way in which you can get rid of these parasites.

How do these parasites occur in your system? Eating unhygienic food, eating food, which has not been washed properly are some of the main factors which encourage the growth of parasites in your tummy and intestinal system. This is a remedy followed for 3 days in a place I know to deparasite kids. 50 g of pomegranate root bark powdered is boiled in 150 g water. When the water is 50 g, it is given to all the kids 1st thing in the morning, for 3 days. On the 4th day, you are going to find all tummy parasites getting eliminated.

Diarrhea

Diarrhea is a really scary sort of ailment, which can rapidly become life-threatening, especially when you do not find any way to stop it. That is because the essential minerals and nutrients of the body are all eliminated. So if you do not have immediate access to medical aid or oral hydration solution, make up a powder of equal amounts of coriander, cumin seed, and aniseed. Drink this with pomegranate juice.

You can also mash one ripe banana in pomegranate juice. Or add 2 teaspoons full of mint leaves juice to pomegranate juice, warm it up to lukewarm temperature and drink it down. There, you have 3 remedies, right at hand, when someone in the family has started to suffer from diarrhea, and the doctor is far, far away.

Gastric Problems

Are you suffering from gastric problems? This normally occurs, when you eat food, which is difficult to digest, especially meat products. Try this remedy to cure gastric problems – one pinch of black salt, hundred grams of pomegranate seeds, 5 g of aniseed and bishops weed, 3 g of cumin seeds. Make up a mixture of these spices with lemon juice, to make a chutney. This delicious chutney needs to be eaten with your lunch and dinner. Not only is this going to solve your gastric problems, but it is also going to help in proper digestion.

Nausea

Nausea is normally caused when you have not been eating hygienic food, or you have overeaten spicy, rich and fatty fried foods. I gave you the recipe of a churna a little while ago. Give the patient two or 3 of these beans to suck. This is going to make the feeling of nausea disappear. He may ask for more, because they are so tasty. Allow him to have 2 or 3 more after an hour or so.

Pomegranate digestive chutney

Here is another tasty chutney which you can make especially when you know that all the people at your party are going to overeat on rich and spicy food. Green coriander, mint, black salt, pepper, and pomegranate seeds, in proportions you like along with one clove. Put them all in a blender and grind. Encourage your guests to eat this chutney, so that they do not suffer from nausea, constipation and indigestion brought about by gorging rich and spicy dishes.

Constipation

The problem with constipation is the amount of side effects it has especially feeling lethargic, lazy, pain in the tummy, and headache. If the constipation is chronic, it can give rise to even more serious ailments. So the 1st thing to prevent constipation is to eat plenty of fresh fruit and vegetables. Drink pomegranate juice as often as you can, after eating a spoonful of bishops weed. For people suffering from chronic constipation, this is a remedy, which is been in use for millenniums. You need a copper utensil for this.

Using Copper Utensils

These are very common in the East, though they are going out of vogue [or need to come in vogue] in the West. Just place fresh water in a copper utensil, leave it covered throughout the day, and drink it at night. The next morning, you are going to find your system cleared and your constipation gone with the wind, no pun intended. This is the reason why people in the East, do not suffer from chronic constipation. The water utensils placed by the side of their beds are made out of copper, and they drink this water, whenever they wake up during the night.

Sugarcane juice remedy

I also found this really effective, especially in the summer, where I have easy access to sugarcane juice. Sugarcane juice with lemon, is one of the most popular nourishing and refreshing summer drinks in the East. I ask the juice vendor whether he can put some pomegranate juice in it. Try this with black salt and pepper sprinkled over the juice. Believe me, this drink is addictive. It is known to prevent jaundice in the summer. It is going to keep you well hydrated. It is also going to refresh you miraculously, especially when you have been doing a lot of walking in the sun.

I normally ask our friendly neighborhood sugarcane juice vendor to make up 3 glasses of sugarcane juice every morning, which I place in the fridge. Then during the day, I mix other fruit juices, like carrot juice, lemon juice, and pomegranate juice in this mixture, and drink this. Believe me, this is an amazing antioxidant and the best thing is that this does wonders to your skin. Try this remedy next summer and be happy that you are getting fresh juices in you!

Excess of Salivation

All right, this is a remedy for an ailment which may sound hilarious, but it troubles a lot of us. Access salivation, due to a problem in the salivary glands. This normally occurs in children, and believe me, both I and my brother suffered from it, when we were kids. We were immediately put onto a no sugar diet and I am not very sure whether that was responsible for making us stop drooling like our pet Cocker Spaniel. Nevertheless, sometimes I find myself with access of saliva in my mouth, especially while I am talking. This remedy was given to me by my friendly neighborhood shaman, who, at the age of 60 prevented salivation from troubling him, because of an infection in his salivary glands.

Warm some pomegranate juice. Now, roast some alum on a griddle, and powder it into a fine powder. Mix this powder into the pomegranate juice. Put this mixture into warm water and gargle and rinse your mouth with this mouthwash. It is going to get rid of all that excess saliva collecting in your mouth. This salivation normally occurs, when you are dehydrated. So drink plenty of fresh juice.

You can also get rid of salivation by roasting sunbaked pomegranate peelss on a fire. When they are shriveled up and brown, powder them. Do not allow them to turn into ashes! Now put a little bit of this powder in half a teaspoonful of honey. Eat it once a day or whenever you feel that saliva production in your mouth is getting out of hand.

Also, I have found that if I eat pomegranate seeds, ginger, lemon and bishops weed along with my meals, I do not find myself suffering from saliva. Well, the food has been digested well, and I do not need to spit out that excess saliva ever so often. You may want to get your throat checked by a proper doctor to see if there is some infection in that area, which is causing this salivation.

Hot foods

You can also try avoiding eating nonvegetarian and high-protein foods especially in the Summers like fish, chicken, too many mangoes eggs, spices, ginger and garlic, dried fruit and nuts. These encourage you to salivate more. On the other hand, these foods are eaten, more in winter, because they are considered to be heat producing.

Suffering from a sore throat?

This normally happens when you eat something sour, no pun intended, or something extremely cold, cough, cold, and other winter related diseases. Now you have some really interesting remedies, with which you can get rid of sore throats, especially in the winter.

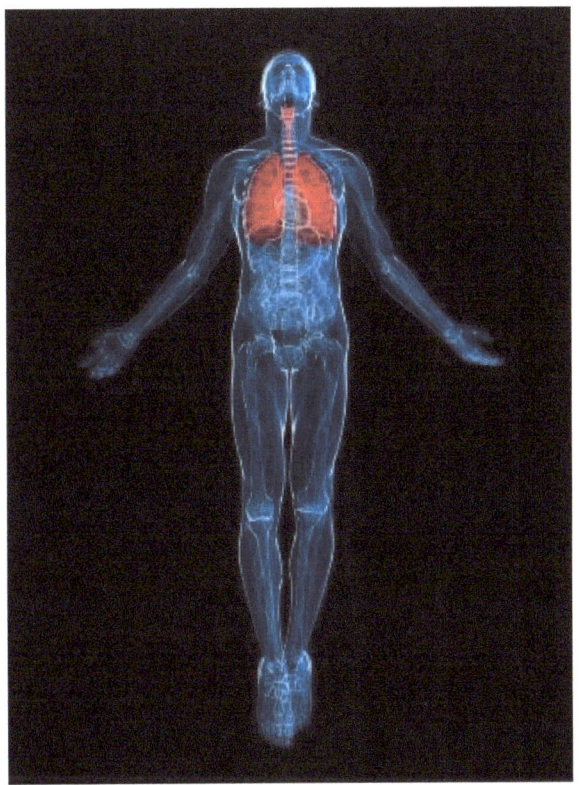

A continuous sore throat may be a symptom of infections in your chest region.

Alum has a tendency to lose its crystalline form when it is heated. It becomes a powder. This heated alum powder is extremely useful in making up a lot of natural recipes. So remember that any time you need to make up a recipe calling for alum powder, do not powder it straight from its crystalline form. Heat it, and then powder it. This is more powerful.

Add 2 teaspoons pomegranate juice to a glass of warm water. Add a little bit of heated powder alum to this mixture. I also use salt in this water to prevent any throat infections. Gargle with it, morning and evening to get rid of that sore throat.

In the same manner, make a powder of sun-dried pomegranate peelss. Sun drying means drying the skins in a shady corner of your sunny porch, in the fresh air. I normally sun dry the skins along with the skins of other fruit. They are excellent as powdered beauty pack ingredients. I normally keep waiting for summer, because with the plethora of so many summer fruits, I have plenty of rinds and skins to add to my collection of herbal remedy and beauty pack ingredients.

Take one spoon of powdered pomegranate peelss and one spoon of powdered licorice. Make up a mixture and add this to a glass of warm water. Keep gargling as often as possible with this mixture. You can also drink it, because licorice, as well as pomegranate are healthy and keep your system functioning properly, both internally and externally.

Nosebleed

This is a recipe, which I found after 20 years – it had been lost in my collected files. My grandmother used it for me, when I used to suffer from nosebleeds as a child. So here it is. If you are suffering from nosebleed, especially in the summer, – which may come of eating hot foods and in the summer heat – cool down the system immediately by drinking one spoon of pomegranate juice with one spoon of gooseberry juice. She also made me drink pomegranate sherbet to prevent me from suffering from sunstroke, because I was a sun worshiper and could not be made to stay indoors, even in the hot summer heat of South and West India.

Pomegranate sherbet

Drink this regularly in the summer, especially if you are living in a region when the sun shines bright and brassy throughout the day. Take 250 g of juice made up of fresh pomegranate seeds. Place this juice in the sun for a little while, so that it can manage to assimilate the goodness of the sun and the fresh air. Now add 2 pinches of heated alum in 2 kg of sugar. Put on heat with a little bit of pomegranate juice, in order to melt the sugar. Now add the rest of the juice and allow it to cook on slow heat until it boils twice. This should not take more than 4 to 5 minutes, depending on the heat. Allow it to cool. This is your pomegranate sherbet which you are going to drink in the ratio of 4 teaspoons sherbet to one glass of iced water.

This is considered to be a great coolant, antioxidant, and also prevents dehydration. Also, you are not going to suffer from any mineral deficiency in the summer through sweating if you drink this regularly. This is also said to prevent summer skin ailments like to eczema, pimples, and even dry itchy skin. Believe it or not, somebody recommended this sherbet to me to get rid of the dark circles around my eyes, and I tried it out. I guess, the dark circles got removed, when I began to go to bed early and to add more green leafy vegetables to my diet, but this sherbet helped because I knew that my body was getting detoxified and I was drinking something healthy. So no more panda eyes, baby!

It seems, drinking this sherbet regularly for 3 months is going to regulate your system so that you may find yourself cured of many chronic problems. Well, I did not have the patience to try out this experiment, because 1] I do not suffer from many chronic diseases, yet, and 2] I would rather drink this as a refreshing drink than as a medicine! So I just drink this in the summer, especially when I have to go out.

Urinary problems

Do you find yourself wanting to void your urinary bladder too many times during the day. This happens sometimes when you have drunk hot water, too much of hot liquids like tea and coffee, and even if you find yourself getting soaked in the rain. Old people suffer from this problem because of age-related weakness of the urinary bladder system.

Roast pomegranate peelss on a griddle until they are shriveled. Now add 20 g of bishops weed to 50 g of this powder. Eat half a teaspoon of this powder twice a day with warm water.

Pomegranate dates chutney

This is a chutney of which you are going to eat a teaspoon 3 times a day – 25 g pomegranate seeds, 5 peppercorns, 5 raisins, 1 peeled date and four pistachio nuts. This is going to strengthen your urinary system and prevent urinary problems.

Bedwetting

Dates are, of course, the best way to get rid of urinary inconsistency, especially in older people and also those children, who suffer from a bedwetting problem. Feed them a date before they go to sleep and they are going to have a restful night. You may also want to add 2 – 3 dates to their daily diet.

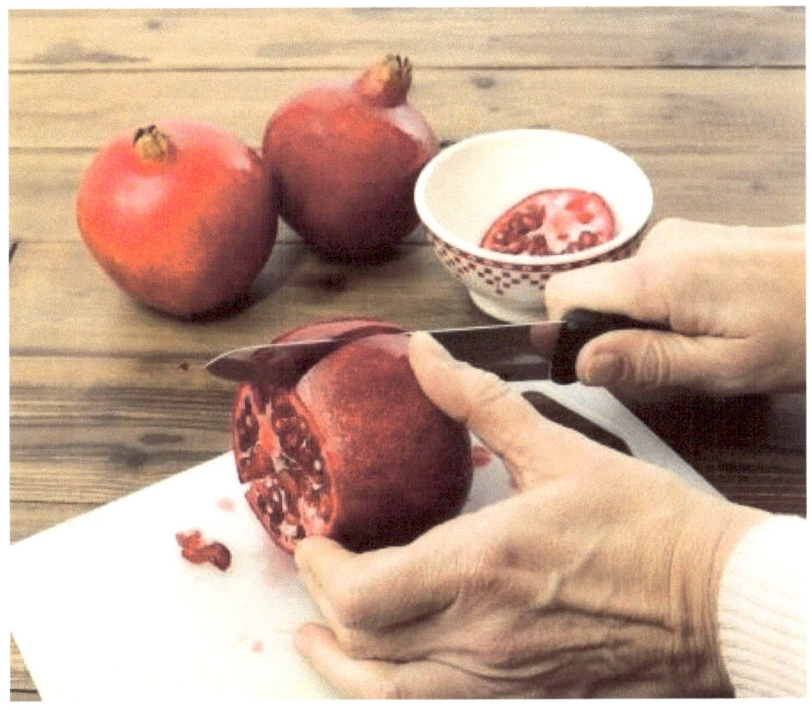

Just rub a little bit of nutmeg in some pomegranate juice, and give to the patient once a day until he is cured completely. You can also make up a mixture of powdered bishops weed sprinkled on half a teaspoonful of fresh pomegranate seeds. This is a tasty teaspoonful which can be given to older children, especially if they still continue bedwetting at the age of 3 or more.

I saw an old grandmother, making up this remedy in the coastal areas of Burma. She just picked out a green unripe banana straight from her garden, and heated it. After that, she added a spoonful of honey and black sesame seeds to the mashed banana. After that, she made small chickpea sized balls of this mixture. All her grandchildren were fed this with pomegranate juice once a day to keep their system right and to prevent any sort of bedwetting.

Conclusion

Well, I have not even touched one 50th of the natural remedies for ailments which can be cured by the not so humble pomegranate. These recipes are taken from ancient Greek, Chinese, Persian, Indian and Egyptian medical books. Most of them are time-tested recipes for common ailments, but all of them acknowledge the fact that pomegranate is a cure-all. So, this book, I hope is going to give you some information about the power of a pomegranate. It is going to keep you healthy, it is going to beautify you, and it is the best antitoxin of which you can dream. So going to your garden and pick up our right pomegranate, right now. Take out its red delicious seeds, sprinkle some rock salt or black salt to add a spicy flavor and savor the taste of crunchy pomegranate ripened in the sun. You may also want to add pomegranate seeds to your salads, especially in the summer. Dried pomegranate seeds are normally made of sour pomegranates and are a very spicy addition to Eastern cuisine for millenniums.

So the next time you eat a pomegranate, do not throw its skin or peel away. Cut the fruit with a very sharp knife from stalk top to apex. You can then remove the pomegranate seeds easily. The peel is going to be thick with a white under skin layer. Collect the peels in an airtight box and when you think you have enough of peels along with other citrus fruit peels, and it is a sunny day outside, just place them on a piece of cloth in the shade outdoors. Cover these peels with a muslin cloth or a net cloth, so that they are not contaminated by insects and dust. It takes 2 to 3 days for these peels to dry up really well. Just grind them and place them in glass bottles. And then use them in beauty recipes as well as in healthy remedies of which you have learned in this book of our magic series.So let the power of the pomegranate keep you healthy and beautiful!

Author Bio

Dueep Jyot Singh is a Management and IT Professional who managed to gather Postgraduate qualifications in Management and English and Degrees in Science, French and Education while pursuing different enjoyable career options like being an hospital administrator, IT,SEO and HRD Database Manager/ trainer, movie scriptwriter, theatre artiste and public speaker, lecturer in French, Marketing and Advertising, ex-Editor of Hearts On Fire (now known as Solctice) Books Missouri USA, advice columnist and cartoonist, publisher and Aviation School trainer, ex- moderator on Medico.in, banker, student councilor ,travelogue writer ... among other things! One fine morning, she decided that she had enough of killing herself by Degrees and went back to her first love -- writing. It's more enjoyable! She already has 48 published academic and 14 fiction- in- different- genre books under her belt.

When she is not designing websites or making Graphic design illustrations for clients who want Walt Disney, Norman Rockwell , JJ Grandville or Hed Kandy type illustrations, she is busy browsing in old bookshops for antique books,-she has a mouthwatering collection of priceless First editions and rare books...including R.L. Stevenson, O.Henry, Dornford Yates, Maurice Walsh, C.N.Williamson, and the crown of her collection- Dickens "The Old Curiosity Shop," and so on... Just call her "Renaissance Woman" - collecting herbal remedies, making one of a kind creations in Irish Crochet and Aran knitting, acting like Universal Helping Hand/Agony Aunt, or escaping to her dear mountains for a bit of exploring, collecting herbs and plants , trekking, and rappelling.

Check out some of the other JD-Biz Publishing books

Gardening Series on Amazon

Download Free Books!

http://MendonCottageBooks.com

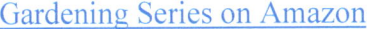

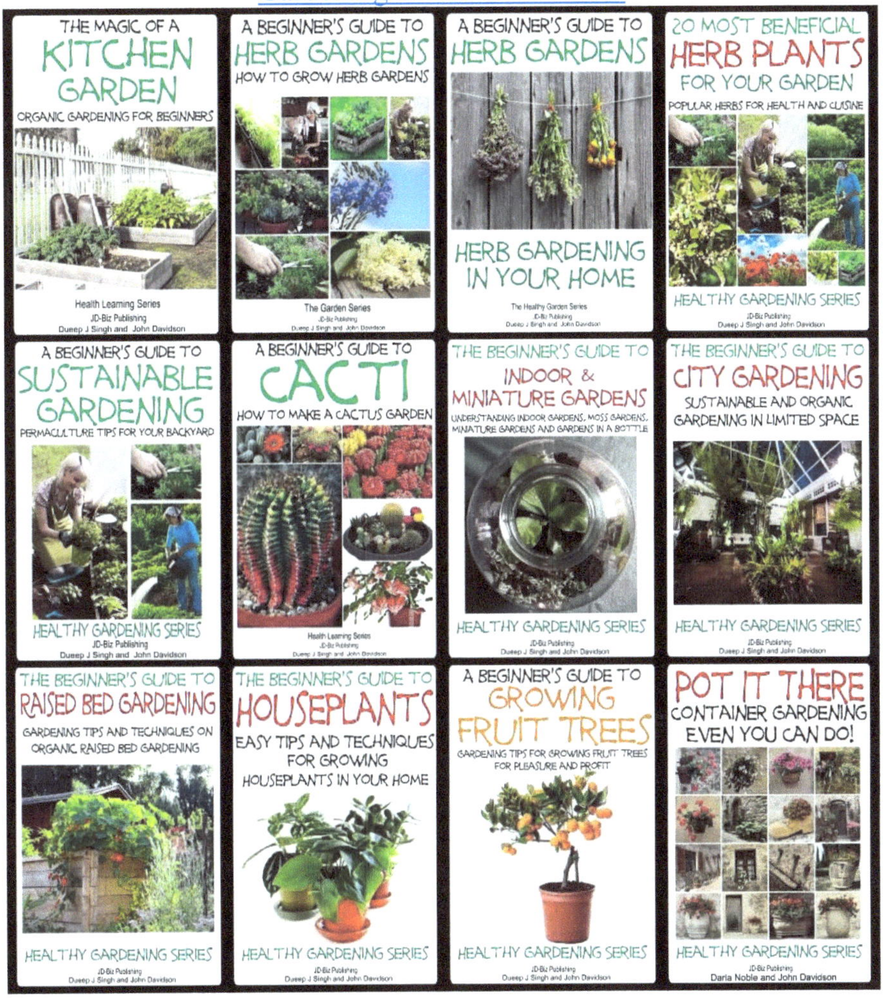

Health Learning Series

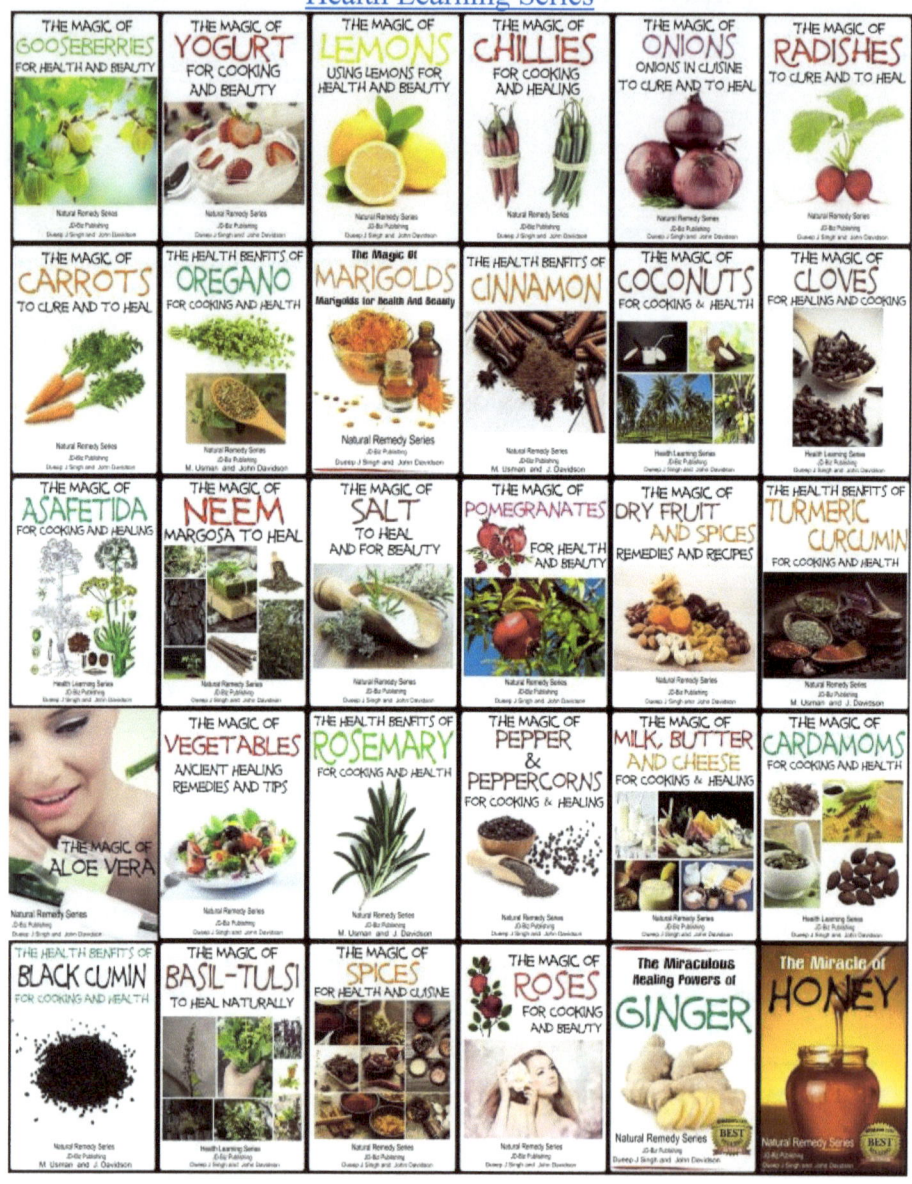

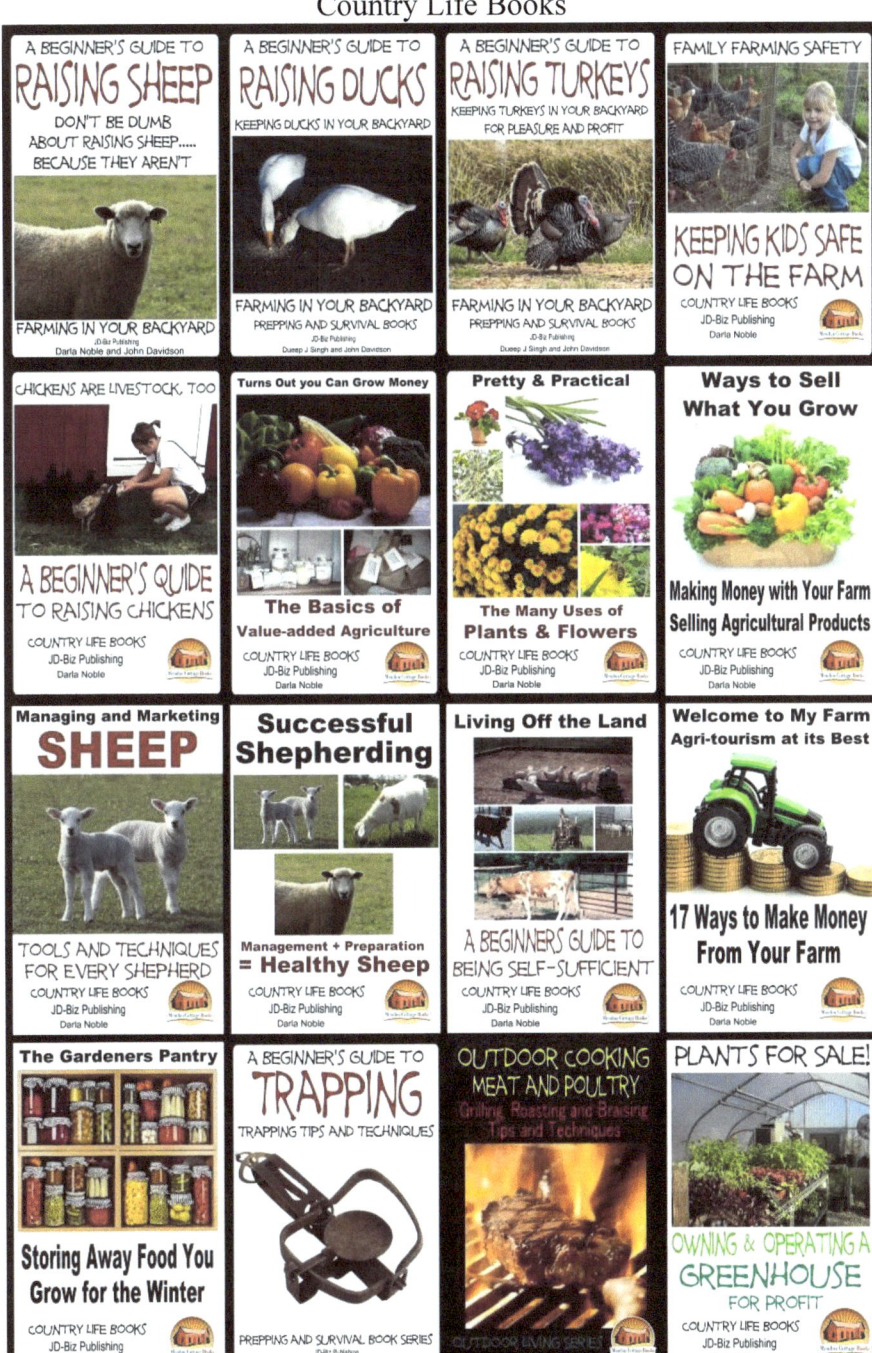

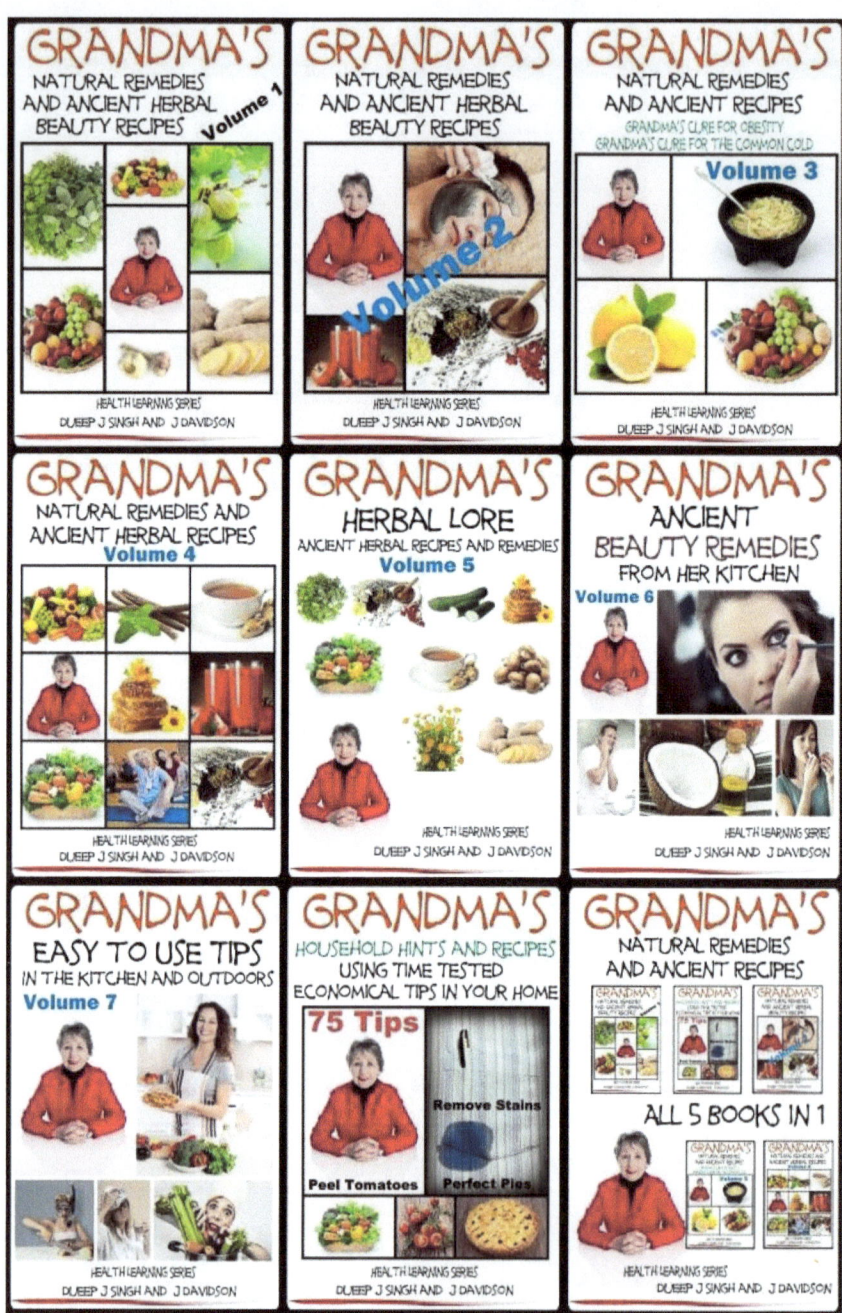

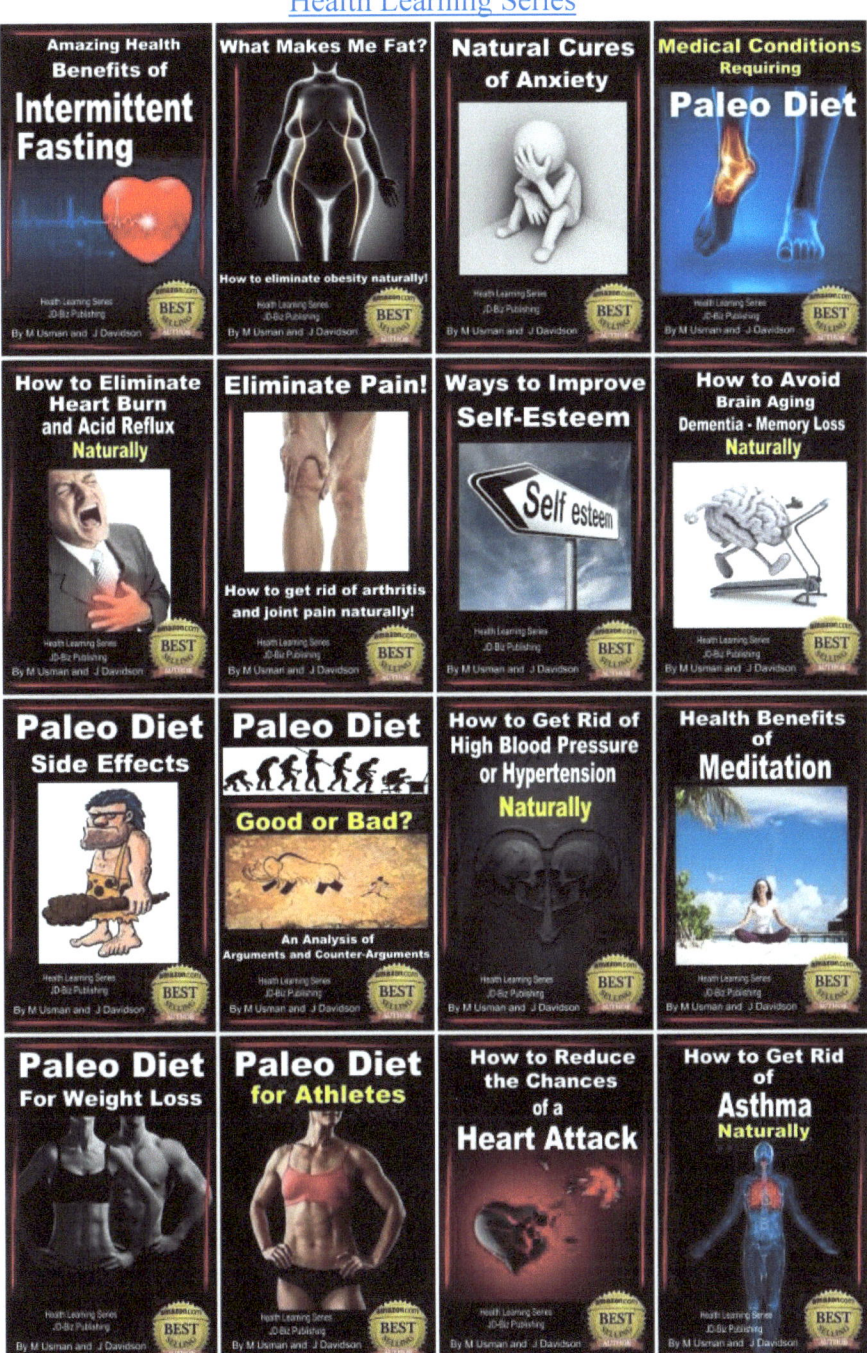

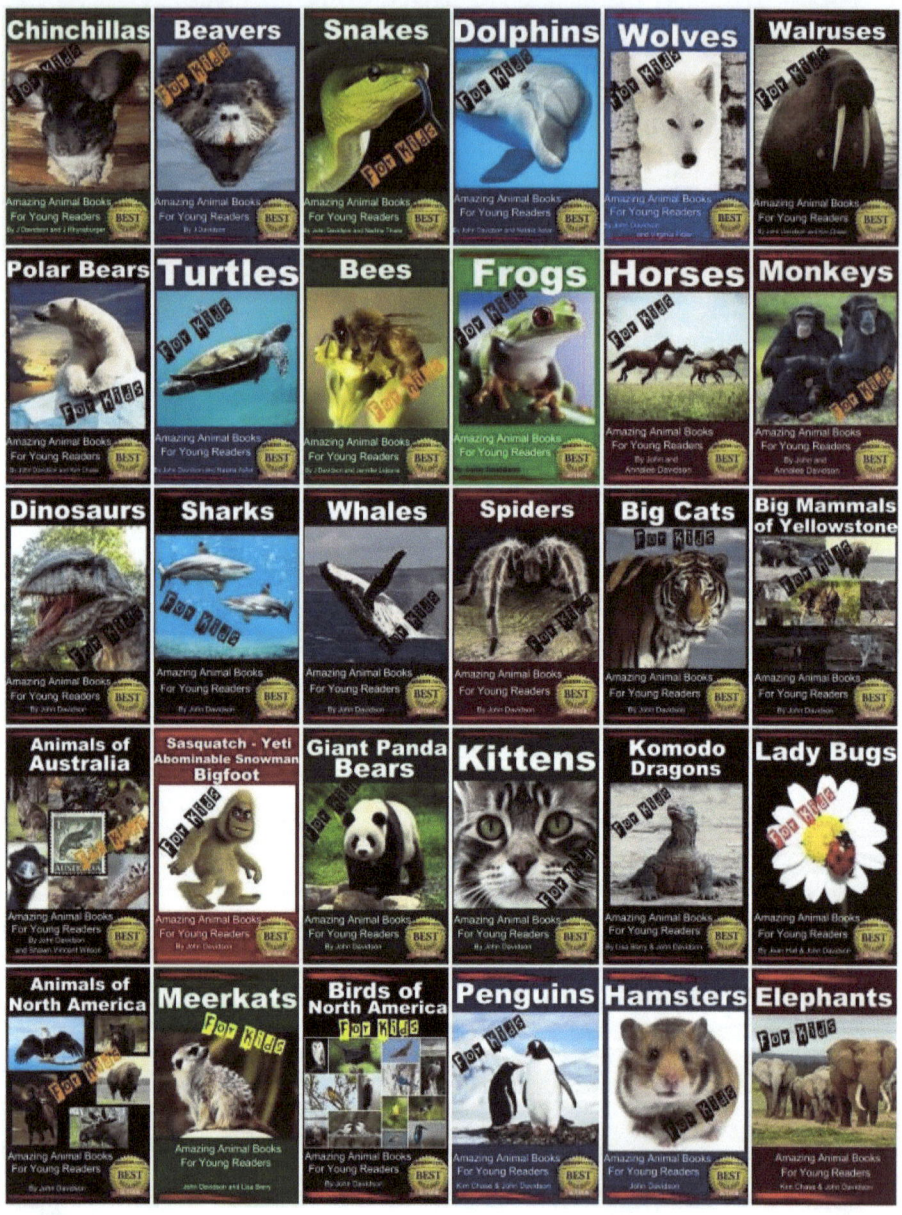

Learn To Draw Series

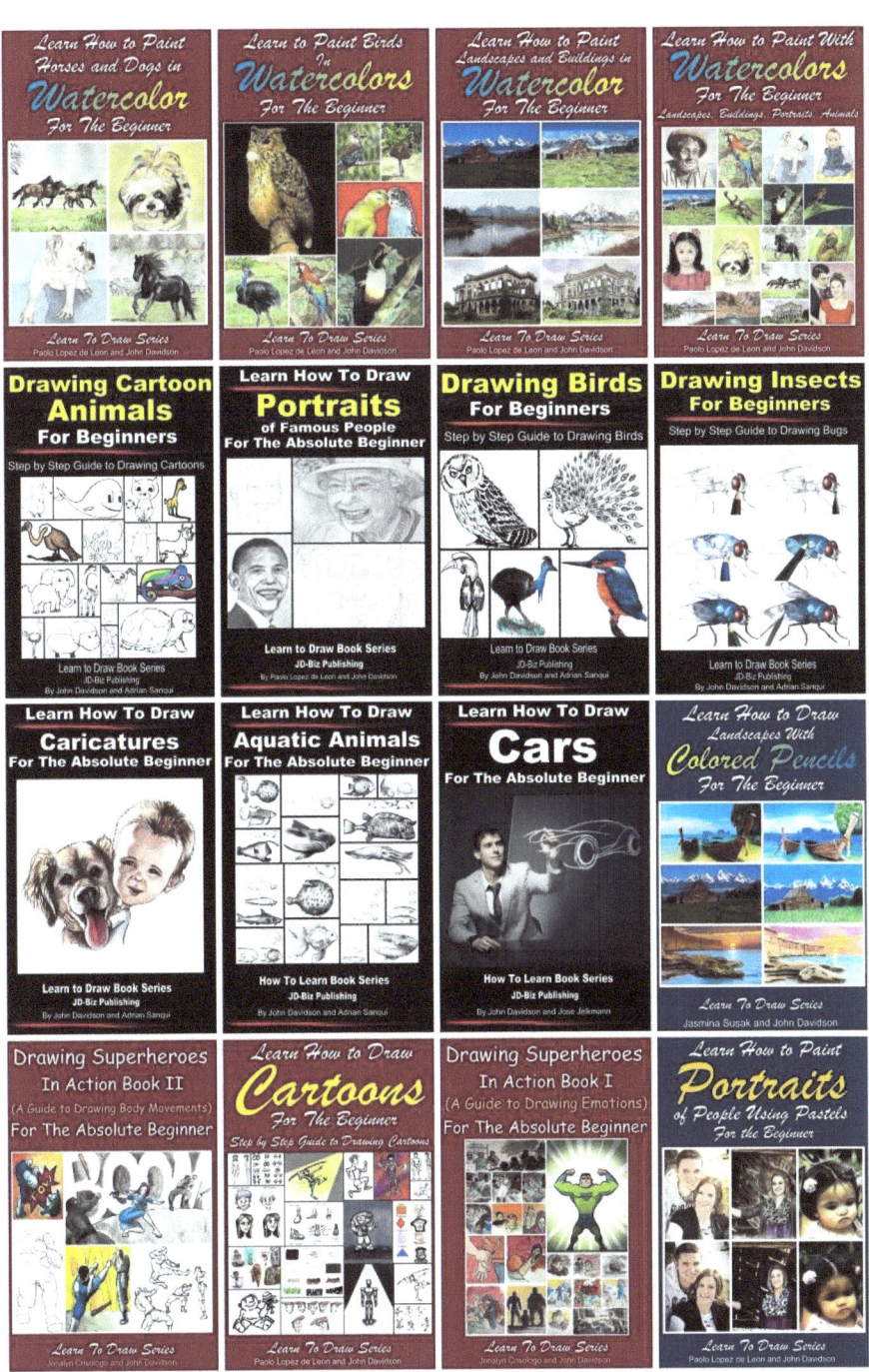

How to Build and Plan Books

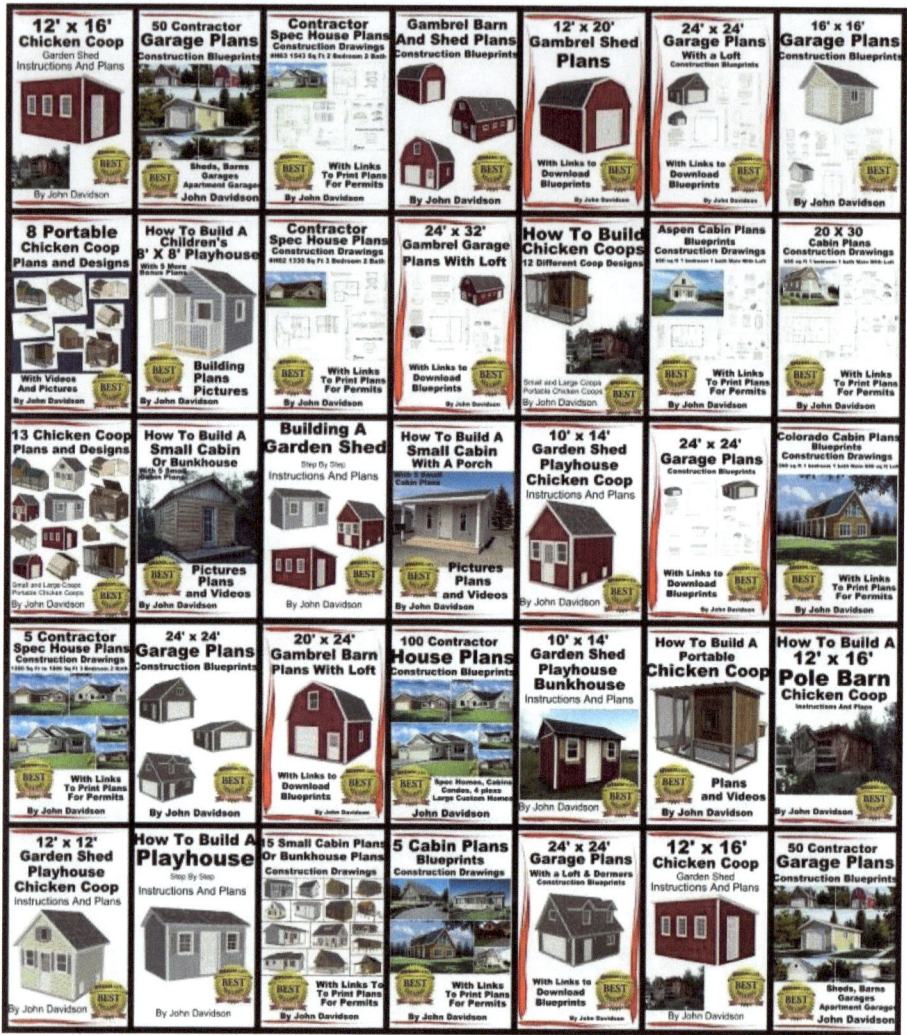

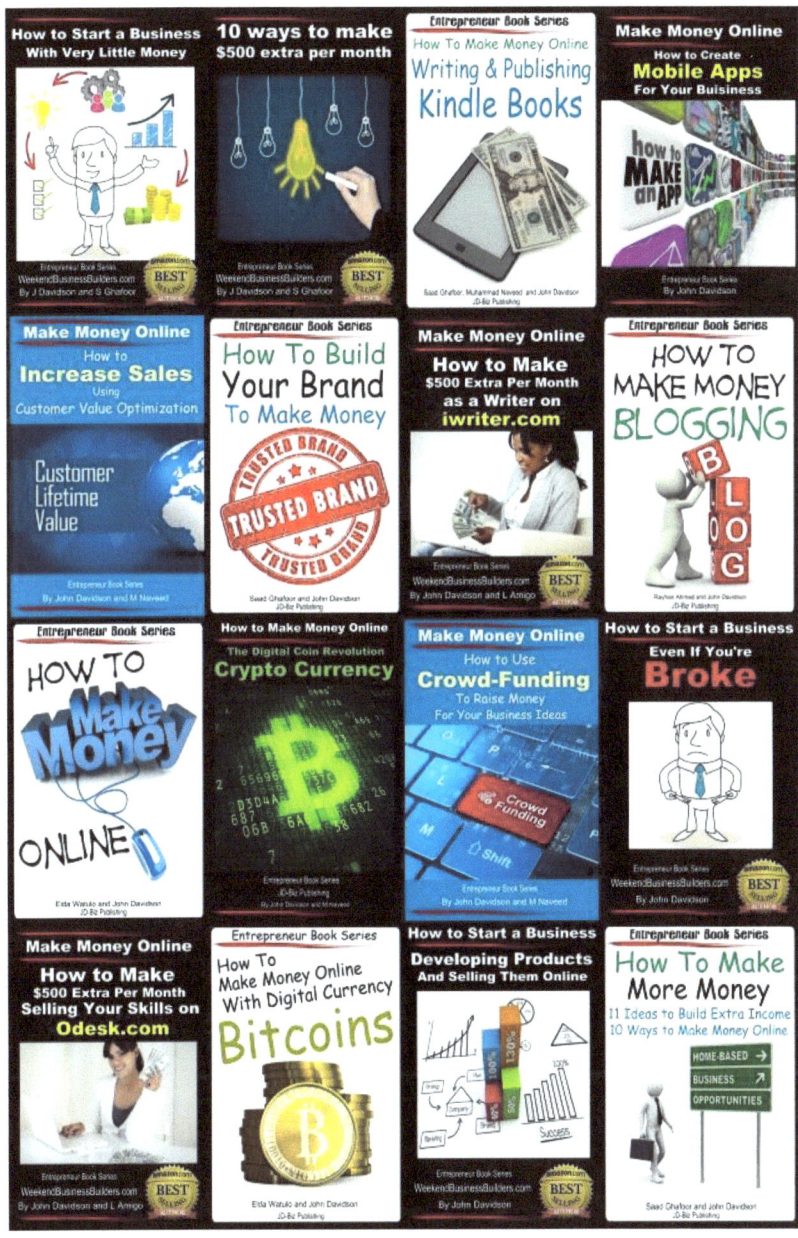

Our books are available at

1. Amazon.com
2. Barnes and Noble
3. Itunes
4. Kobo
5. Smashwords
6. Google Play Books

Download Free Books!

http://MendonCottageBooks.com

Publisher

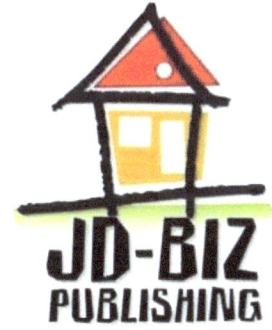

JD-Biz Corp

P O Box 374

Mendon, Utah 84325

http://www.jd-biz.com/

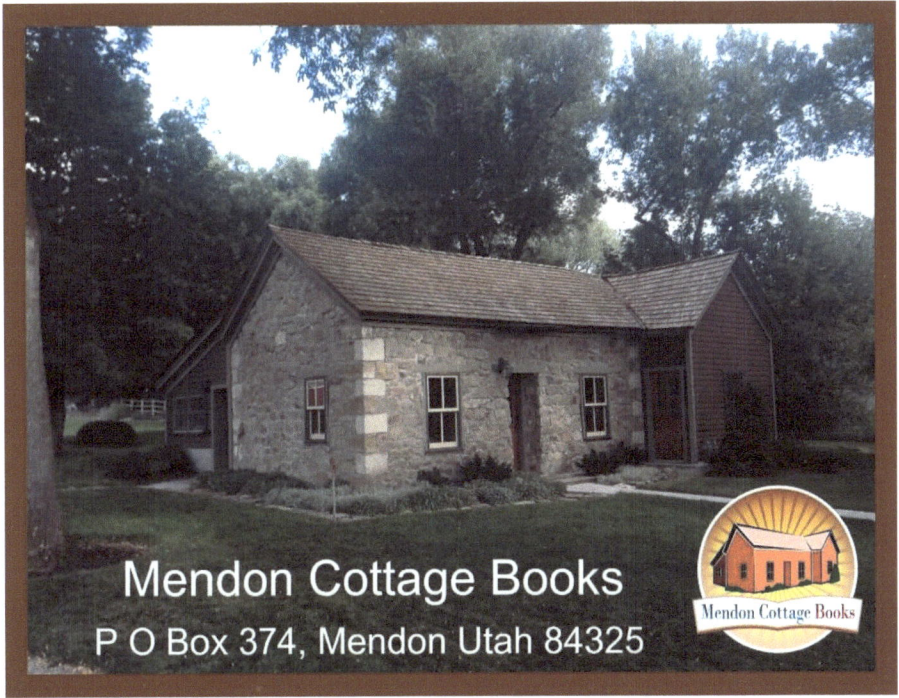